Brief Contents

PART I FOOD SCIENCE AND NUTRITION

1 Food Selection 1
2 Food Evaluation 20
3 Chemistry of Food Composition 27

PART II FOOD SERVICE

4 Food Safety 61
5 Food Preparation Basics 91
6 Meal Management 113

PART III FOODS

PROTEIN—MEAT, POULTRY, FISH, DAIRY, & EGGS

7 Meat 131
8 Poultry 163
9 Fish and Shellfish 177
10 Milk 197
11 Cheese 218
12 Eggs 236

PHYTOCHEMICALS—VEGETABLES, FRUITS, SOUPS, & SALADS

13 Vegetables and Legumes 256
14 Fruits 284
15 Soups, Salads, and Gelatins 310

COMPLEX CARBOHYDRATES—CEREALS, FLOUR, BREADS

16 Cereal Grains and Pastas 326
17 Flours and Flour Mixtures 346
18 Starches and Sauces 369
19 Quick Breads 385
20 Yeast Breads 395

DESSERTS—REFINED CARBOHYDRATES & FAT

21 Sweeteners 411
22 Fats and Oils 428
23 Cakes and Cookies 453
24 Pastries and Pies 471
25 Candy 489
26 Frozen Desserts 505

WATER—BEVERAGES

27 Beverages 518

PART IV FOOD INDUSTRY

28 Food Preservation 541
29 Government Food Regulations 555
30 Careers in Food and Nutrition 570

APPENDIXES

A Food Preparation Equipment A-1
B Food Yields B-1
C Substitution of Ingredients C-1
D Flavorings and Seasonings D-1
E Common Food Additives E-1
F Answers to Multiple-Choice Questions F-1

GLOSSARY G-1
INDEX I-1

Contents

Preface xxiv

About the Author xxvii

PART I FOOD SCIENCE AND NUTRITION

Chapter 1 Food Selection 1

Sensory Criteria 1
Sight 1
Odor 2
Classification of Odors 2
Detecting Odors 2
Taste 3
Mechanism of Taste 3
The Six Taste Stimuli 3
Taste Interactions 4
Factors Affecting Taste 4
Definition of Flavor 4
Touch 4
Hearing 6

Nutritional Criteria 6
Weight Management 6
Dietary Guidelines for Americans 6
ChooseMyPlate 6
SuperTracker 8
Previous Food Group Plans 8
Vegetarianism 8
Consumer Dietary Changes 9
Kcalories on Menus 9
Complementary and Integrative Medicine 9
Functional Foods 10
Nutrigenomics 11

Cultural Criteria 11
Ethnic Influences 11
Place of Birth 11
Geography and Climate 12
Cultural Influences on Manners 12

Religious Criteria 12
Buddhism 12
Hinduism 12
Seventh-Day Adventist Church 12
Church of Jesus Christ of Latter-Day Saints (Mormon Church) 12
Judaism 13
Islam 13

Psychological and Sociological Criteria 14
Bioengineering 14
History of Biotechnology 14
Foods Created with Biotechnology 14
Concerns about GMO Foods 15
Acceptance/Rejection of GM Foods 16
Organic Foods 16
Organic Certification 16
"Natural" Foods 17
Processed Foods 17

Budgetary Criteria 17

Chapter 2 Food Evaluation 20

Sensory (Subjective) Evaluation 20
Two Types of Sensory Testing 20
Analytical (Effective) Tests 22
Affective (Acceptance or Preference) Tests 22
Taste Panels 22
Sample Preparation 23

Objective Evaluation 23
Physical Tests 23
Chemical Tests 24
Electronic Noses 25
Comparison of Sensory and Objective Evaluations 25

Chapter 3 Chemistry of Food Composition 27
Basic Food Chemistry: The Six Key Atoms (CHNOPS) 27
Water 28
Water Content in Foods 29
Composition of Water 29
Measuring Heat Energy 30
Specific Heat 30
Freezing Point 30
Melting Point 31
Boiling Point 31
Elevation and Boiling Point 31
Hard vs. Soft Water 31
Functions of Water in Food 31
Heat Transfer: Moist-Heat Cooking Methods 32
Solvent 32
Dispersions 32
Solutions 33
Colloidal Dispersions 33
Coarse Dispersions (Suspensions) 34
Dispersion Destabilization 34
Chemical Reactions 34
Ionization 34
Changes in pH—Acids and Bases 34
Salt Formation 35
Hydrolysis 35
Carbon Dioxide Release 35
Food Preservation 35
Water Activity 35
Osmosis and Osmotic Pressure 36
Carbohydrates 36
Foods High in Carbohydrates 36
Composition of Carbohydrates 36
Monosaccharides 37
Disaccharides 38
Oligosaccharides 38
Polysaccharides 38
Functions of Carbohydrates in Foods 43
Lipids (Fats) 43
Foods High in Lipids 43
Composition of Lipids 43
Triglycerides 43
Fatty Acids 43
Fatty Acid Structure 43
Fatty Acids in Foods 44
Fatty Acid Nomenclature 45
Phospholipids 45
Food Industry Uses 45
Sterols 45
Plant Sterols 45
Functions of Lipids in Foods 47
Proteins 47
Protein Quality in Foods 47
Composition of Proteins 47
Amino Acids 48
Functions of Proteins in Food 49
Hydration 49
Denaturation/Coagulation 49
Enzymatic Reactions 49
Buffering 51
Browning 51
Vitamins and Minerals 52
Foods High in Vitamins and Minerals 52
Composition of Vitamins and Minerals 53
Functions of Vitamins and Minerals in Food 53
Enrichment and Fortification 53
Antioxidants and Their Food Industry Uses 53
Sodium and Its Food Industry Uses 53
Nonnutritive Food Components 53
Food Additives 54
Purposes of Food Additives 54
Additives that Improve Appeal 54
Additives that Extend Storage Life 56
Additives that Maximize Performance 56
Additives that Protect Nutrient Value 57
Plant Compounds 57
Beneficial 57
Harmful 57
Caffeine 57
PART II FOOD SERVICE
Chapter 4 Food Safety 61
What is a Foodborne Illness? 62
What Causes Foodborne Illness? 62

Biological Hazards—Living Culprits 62
Bacteria: Number-One Cause of Foodborne Illness 63
Food Infections 63
Food Intoxication 64
Toxin-Mediated Infection 64
Bacterial Food Infections 65
Salmonella 65
Listeria monocytogenes 65
Yersinia enterocolitica 65
Shigella 66
Bacterial Food Intoxications 66
Clostridium perfringens 66
Staphylococcus aureus 66
Clostridium botulinum 66
Bacterial Toxin-Mediated Infections 66
Escherichia coli 67
Campylobacter jejuni 68
Vibrio 68
Molds 68
Viruses 68
Hepatitis A Virus 68
Norovirus 69
Parasites 69
Roundworms 69
Protozoa 69
Prions—Mad Cow Disease 70
New Virulent Biological Hazards 71
Advanced Techniques for Detecting Contamination 71
Chemical Hazards—Harmful Chemicals in Food 71
Seafood Toxins: Chemicals from Fish/Shellfish 72
Ciguatera Fish Poisoning 72
Histamine Food Poisoning 73
Puffer Fish Poisoning 73
Red Tide 73
Physical Hazards—Objects in Food 73
Food Allergy, Intolerance, and Sensitivity 73
Allergic Reaction Prevention 73
Labeling of Common Food Allergens 73
Cross-Contamination 73
Preventing Foodborne Illness 74
Prevention Factors Overview 74
Personnel 74
Training 74
Personal Hygiene Habits 74
Food Flow 75
Purchasing: Written Specifications 75
Inspection 76
Storage 76
Temperature 76
Proper Refrigerator and Freezer Use 77
Storage Times 77
Vulnerable Foods 78
High-Risk Foods 78
Foods with High Water Activity 78
Foods with Low Acidity 78
Exceptions to the High-Protein/Water/pH Rules 79
Oxygen and Food 79
Preparation 79
Pre-preparation 79
Cooking (Heating) 80
Holding 80
Proper Use of Thermometers 82
Types of Thermometers 82
Testing Temperatures 82
Care of Thermometers 83
Calibration of Thermometers 83
Cooling 84
Reheating 84
Serving 84
Sanitation 84
Dishes 84
Scheduling 85
Euipment 85
Facilities 85
Pest Control 86
Food Safety Monitoring 86
Health Department Inspections 86
HACCP 87
HARPC 88
Foodborne Illness Surveillance 88
World Health Organization 88

Chapter 5 Food Preparation Basics 91

Heating Foods 91
Moist-Heat Preparation 92

Types of Moist-Heat Preparation 92
Scalding 92
Poaching 92
Simmering 92
Stewing 92
Braising 92
Boiling 93
Steaming 93
Microwaving 93
Dry-Heat Preparation 93

Types of Dry-Heat Preparation 94
Baking 94
- Rack Position 94
- Pan Color 94

Roasting 94
Broiling 94
Grilling 94
Barbecuing 94
Frying 95
- Sautéing and Stir-Frying 95
- Pan-Broiling and Pan-Frying 95
- Deep-Frying 95

Types of Heat Transfer 95
- Conduction 95
- Convection 96
- Radiation 96
- Induction 96

Measuring Heat 96

Cutlery Techniques 97
Handling Knives 97
Cutting Styles 98

Measuring Ingredients 101
Measuring Weight vs. Volume 101
Using Scales 101
- Metric vs. Nonmetric 101

Selecting the Right Measuring Utensil 101
Using an Accurate Measuring Technique 101
- Liquids 101
- Eggs 102
- Fat 102
- Sugar 102
- Flour 103
- Other Ingredients and Substitutions 103
- Approximating Food Requirements 103

Mixing Techniques 104
Baked Products 104

Seasonings and Flavorings 104
Types of Seasonings and Flavorings 104
- Salt 104
- Salt Substitutes 106
- Pepper 106
- Herbs and Spices 106
- Flavor Enhancers 108
- Oil Extracts 108
- Marinades 108
- Rubs and Pastes 108
- Breadings 109
- Batters 109
- Condiments 110

Adding Seasonings and Flavorings to Food 110
- How Much to Add? 110
- When to Add? 110
- Food Industry Uses 110

Chapter 6 Meal Management 113

Food-Service Organization 113
Commercial Food-Service Organization 114
- Escoffier's System of Organization via Stations 114
- Administrative Positions 115

Hospital Food-Service Organization 115

Types of Meal Planning 116
USDA Menu Patterns 116
Hospital Menu Patterns 117
Types of Menus 117
- Cycle Menus 117
- Nutrition 118

Purchasing 118
Buyers 121
Food Stores and Vendors/Suppliers 121
- Supermarkets 122
- Warehouse Stores 122

Co-ops 122
Smaller Outlets 122
Food-Service Vendors 122
Cost Control 122
Meats 122
Fish 122
Dairy 122
Bread/Grains 122
Fruits and Vegetables 122
Price Comparisons 122
Reading Label Product Codes 123
Reducing Waste Saves Costs 123
As Purchased vs. Edible Portion 123
Percentage Yield 123
Portion Control 123

Time Management 124
Estimating Time 124
Efficient Meal Preparation 124
Recipes 124

Types of Meal Service 125
Russian Service 125
French Service 127
English Service 127
American Service 127
Family Service 127
Buffet Service 127

Table Settings 127
Cover and Linens 127
Flatware/Dinnerware/Glassware 127
Accessories 127
Centerpieces 128

PART III FOODS

Chapter 7 Meat 131

Types Of Meats 131
Beef 131
Veal 132
Lamb and Mutton 132
Pork 132

Composition of Meats 132
Structure of Meat 132
Muscle Tissue 132
Connective Tissue 133
Adipose (Fatty) Tissue 133
Bone 134
Antibiotics and Hormones 134
Pigments 136
Effect of Oxygen on Color 136
Effect of Heat on Color 137
Extractives 137

Purchasing Meats 137
Inspection 137
Grading 139
Quality 139
Yield 140
Tenderness of Meats 141
Natural Tenderizing 141
Artificial Tenderizing 143
Cuts of Meat 144
Terminology of Retail Cuts 144
Beef Retail Cuts 144
Veal Retail Cuts 146
Pork Retail Cuts 146
Lamb Retail Cuts 147
Variety Meats 147
Kosher Meats 149
Halal Meats 149
Organic Meats 149
Processed Meats 149
Processing Methods 149
Food Additives in Processed Meats 150
Types of Processed Meat 152
Mechanically Deboned Meat 152
Restructured Meat 153

Preparation Of Meats 153
Changes during Heating 153
Tenderness and Juiciness 153
Searing 153
Flavor Changes 154
Flavor Enhancements 154
Determining Doneness 154
Internal Temperature 154
Time/Weight Charts 155
Color Changes 155
Touch 156
Dry-Heat Preparation 156
Roasting 156
Broiling and Grilling 156

Pan-Broiling 157
Frying 157
Deep-Frying 158
Moist-Heat Preparation 158
Braising 158
Simmering or Stewing 158
Steaming 159
Microwaving 159
Carving 159

Storage of Meats 159
Refrigerated 159
Wrapping Meat 159
Refrigeration Times 159
Packaging 160
Frozen 160

Chapter 8 Poultry 163

Classification of Poultry 163

Composition of Poultry 163

Purchasing Poultry 163
Inspection 163
Grading 165
Types and Styles of Poultry 165
Processed Poultry 165
Labeling 166
Standardized Poultry Buying 166
How Much to Buy 167

Preparation of Poultry 168
Preparation Safety Tips 168
Thawing Frozen Poultry 168
Stuffing 168
Brining 168
Changes during Preparation 169
Determining Doneness 170
Internal Temperature 170
Color Change 170
Touch 170
Time/Weight Charts 170
Dry-Heat Preparation 170
Roasting or Baking 170
Broiling or Grilling 172
Frying 173
Moist-Heat Preparation 173
Braising 173
Stewing 173
Poaching 173
Microwaving 173

Storage of Poultry 174
Refrigerated 174
Frozen 174

Chapter 9 Fish and Shellfish 177

Classification of Fish and Shellfish 177
Vertebrate or Invertebrate 177
Vertebrates 178
Invertebrates 178
Saltwater or Freshwater 178
Lean or Fat 178

Composition of Fish 178
Structure of Finfish 178
Collagen 179
Amino Acid Content 179
Muscle Structure 179
Pigments 179

Purchasing Fish and Shellfish 180
Inspection/Grading 181
Shellfish Certification 181
Selection of Finfish 181
Fresh and Frozen Fish 181
Canned Fish 184
Cured Fish 185
Fabricated Fish 185
Caviar 186
Selection of Shellfish 186
Purchasing Live Shellfish 186
Purchasing Processed Shellfish 187
Shucking Shellfish 187
Oysters 187
Clams 188
Scallops 188
Mussels 188
Abalone 188
Lobsters 188
Shrimp 189
Crab 189
Crayfish 190

Preparation of Fish and Shellfish 190
Dry-Heat Preparation 190

Baking 190
Broiling 191
Grilling 191
Frying 191
Moist-Heat Preparation 191
Poaching 191
Simmering 192
Steaming 192
Microwaving 192
Raw Fish Preparation 193
Sashimi 193
Sushi 193
Ceviche 193
Food Safety Concerns 193

Storage of Fish and Shellfish 193
Fresh Finfish 194
Refrigerated 194
Spoilage Factors 194
Storing Caviar 194
Fresh Shellfish 194
Frozen 194
Thawing 194
Canned and Cured 194

Chapter 10 Milk 197

Functions of Milk in Foods 198

Composition of Milk 198
Nutrients 198
Carbohydrate 198
Protein 199
Fat 199
Vitamins 200
Minerals 200
Color Compounds 200
Food Additives 201

Purchasing Milk 202
Grades 202
Pasteurization 202
Ultrapasteurization 202
Ultrahigh-Temperature Processing 202
Homogenization 203

Types of Milk 204
Fresh Fluid Cow Milks 204
Whole Milk 204
Reduced-Fat and Low-Fat Milks 204
Fat-Free or Nonfat Milk 204
Fresh Fluid Milks from Other Animals 204
Flavored Fluid Milks 204
Chocolate Milk 205
Eggnog 205
Ultrahigh-Temperature Milk (UHT) 205
Nutritionally Altered Fluid Milks 205
Imitation Milk 206
Filled Milk 206
Low-Sodium Milk 206
Reduced-Lactose Milk 206
Plant-Based "Milks" 206
Soy Milk 206
Rice Milk 206
Almond Milk 206
Nut Milks 207
Hemp Milk 207
Grain Milk 207
Coconut Milk 207
Canned Fluid Milks 207
Whole Milk 207
Evaporated Milk 207
Sweetened Condensed Milk 208
Dry Milk 208
Nonfat Dry Milk 208
Instant Milk 208
Cultured Milk Products 208
Cultures Added to Milk 208
Buttermilk 209
Yogurt 210
Functional Foods—Probiotics 211
Acidophilus Milk 211
Kefir 211
Sour Cream 211
Creams and Substitutes 212
Cream 212
Cream Substitutes 212

Milk Products in Food Preparation 212
Flavor Changes 212
Coagulation and Precipitation 212
Heat 212
Acid 212
Enzymes 213
Salts 213
Whipped Milk Products 213

Whipped Cream 213
Whipped Evaporated Milk 214
Whipped Reconstituted Nonfat Dry Milk 215

Storage of Milk Products 215
Refrigerated 215
Dry Storage 215

Chapter 11 Cheese 218

Classification of Cheeses 218
Place of Origin 219
Moisture Content 219

Cheese Production 219
Milk Selection 221
Coagulation 221
Enzyme Coagulation 221
Acid Coagulation 223
Curd Treatment 223
Curing and Ripening 224
Whey and Whey Products 226
Whey Cheeses 228
Dry Whey 228
Modified Whey Products 228
Process (Processed) Cheeses 228
Process Cheese 228
Cold-Pack Cheese 228
Process Cheese Food 229
Process Cheese Spread 229
Imitation Cheese 229
Tofu and Other Nondairy Cheeses 229
Food Additives in Cheese 229

Purchasing Cheese 229
Grading 229
Forms of Cheese 230

Food Preparation with Cheese 230
Selecting a Cheese 230
Shreddability 230
Meltability 230
Oiling Off 231
Blistering 231
Browning 231
Stretchability 231
Temperatures 231
Cutting Cheese 232

Storage of Cheese 232
Dry Storage 232
Refrigeration 232
Frozen 233

Chapter 12 Eggs 236

Composition of Eggs 236
Yolk 236
Albumen 237
Shell Membranes 237
Air Cell 237
Shell 238

Purchasing Eggs 238
Inspection 238
Eggs Failing USDA Inspection 238
Grading 238
Grading Methods 238
Sizing 240
Egg Substitutes 240
Value-Added Eggs 240

Types of Eggs 241

Functions of Eggs in Foods 241
Emulsifying 241
Binding 241
Foaming 241
Beating Technique 243
Temperature 243
Bowl Selection 244
Separation of Eggs 244
Additives 244
Interfering 244
Clarifying 244
Color 244

Preparation of Eggs 244
Changes in Prepared Eggs 245
Effects of Temperature and Time 245
Effects of Added Ingredients 245
Color Changes 245
Dry-Heat Preparation 246
Frying 246
Baking 247
Moist-Heat Preparation 248
Hard or Soft "Boiling" 248
Coddling 249
Poaching 249

Custards 250
Microwaving 250

Storage of Eggs 251
Refrigerator 251
Whole Eggs 251
Storage Eggs 251
Pasteurized Eggs 251
Frozen 251
Dried 252
Rehydrating Dried Eggs 252
Safety Tips 252
Purchase 253
Preparation 253
Consumption 253
Storage 253

Chapter 13 Vegetables and Legumes 256

Classification of Vegetables 256

Composition of Vegetables 256
Structure of Plant Cells 256
Cell Wall 256
Storage Structures in Parenchyma Cells 257
Intercellular Air Spaces 258
Plant Pigments 258
Carotenoids 258
Chlorophyll 258
Flavonoids 259
Plants as Functional Foods 259
Additives 261

Purchasing Vegetables 263
Grading Vegetables 263
Selecting Vegetables 263
Artichoke 263
Asparagus 266
Beans (Green Snap, Green, Wax, and Yellow Wax-Pod Beans) 266
Beets 266
Broccoli 266
Brussels Sprouts 266
Cabbage 266
Carrots 266
Cauliflower 266
Celery 266
Corn 266
Cucumbers 266
Eggplant 267
Exotic Vegetables 267
Garlic 267
Ginger 268
Greens 268
Leeks 268
Lettuce 268
Mushrooms 268
Okra 269
Onions 269
Parsley 270
Parsnips 270
Peas 270
Peppers, Hot 270
Peppers, Sweet 270
Potatoes 270
Radishes 271
Rutabagas 271
Spinach 271
Sprouts 271
Squash 272
Sweet Potatoes 272
Tomatoes 273
Turnips 273

Legumes 273
Textured Vegetable Protein 274
Meat Analogs 274
Tofu 274
Fermented Soybean Foods 274

Preparation of Vegetables 275
General Guidelines 275
Changes During Heating 275
Texture 275
Flavor 275
Odor 276
Color 276
Nutrient Retention 277
Dry-Heat Preparation 277
Baking 277
Roasting 278
Frying 278
Moist-Heat Preparation 278
Simmering 278